YOUR KNOWLEDGE HAS VALUE

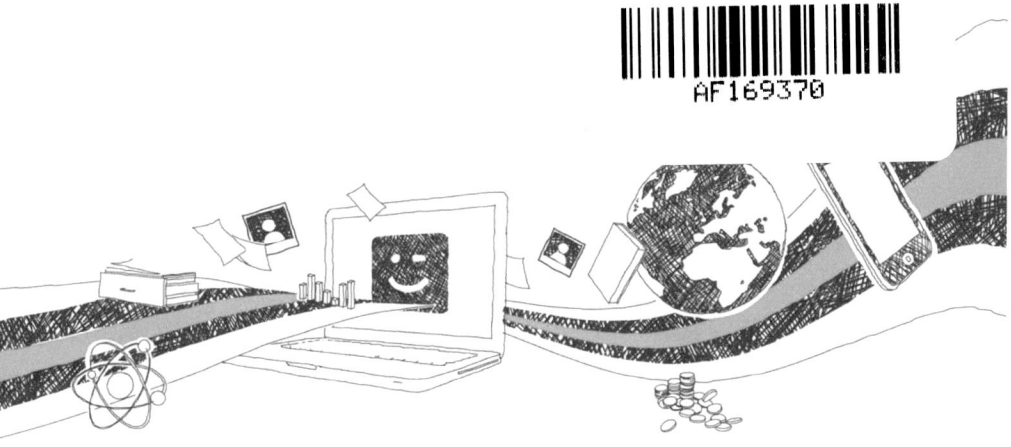

- We will publish your bachelor's and master's thesis, essays and papers

- Your own eBook and book - sold worldwide in all relevant shops

- Earn money with each sale

Upload your text at www.GRIN.com
and publish for free

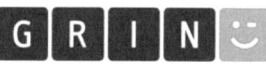

Bibliographic information published by the German National Library:

The German National Library lists this publication in the National Bibliography; detailed bibliographic data are available on the Internet at http://dnb.dnb.de .

This book is copyright material and must not be copied, reproduced, transferred, distributed, leased, licensed or publicly performed or used in any way except as specifically permitted in writing by the publishers, as allowed under the terms and conditions under which it was purchased or as strictly permitted by applicable copyright law. Any unauthorized distribution or use of this text may be a direct infringement of the author s and publisher s rights and those responsible may be liable in law accordingly.

Imprint:

Copyright © 2016 GRIN Verlag, Open Publishing GmbH
Print and binding: Books on Demand GmbH, Norderstedt Germany
ISBN: 9783668479630

This book at GRIN:

http://www.grin.com/en/e-book/368340/social-media-and-nursing-how-the-use-of-social-media-affects-the-health

Leonard Kahungu

Social Media and Nursing. How the Use of Social Media affects the Health Care Sector

GRIN Publishing

GRIN - Your knowledge has value

Since its foundation in 1998, GRIN has specialized in publishing academic texts by students, college teachers and other academics as e-book and printed book. The website www.grin.com is an ideal platform for presenting term papers, final papers, scientific essays, dissertations and specialist books.

Visit us on the internet:

http://www.grin.com/

http://www.facebook.com/grincom

http://www.twitter.com/grin_com

Sociological Theoretical Approach
Leonard Kahungu

Summaries of the Findings 2
Sociological Theoretical Approach 4
References 8

Summaries of the Findings

The modern technology has revolutionized the industrial sectors in unique ways. The incorporation of the contemporary technology significantly affects the health care system is various ways. As a consequence, the efficiency of the overall system has extensively improved. Unfortunately, the integration of these developments leads to a number of challenges.

Particularly, the use of social media in nursing platforms plays a central role in enhancing the communication techniques and reaching a wider geographical region within a short period at relatively reduced costs. Enrico Coiera explores the use of social media and how it affects the health care sector. Communication methods are changing due to the growth of technology. Thus, the nursing community must establish the appropriate ways to include social media. Social media has the capacity to foster the relationship between the nurse community and other health care organizations to enhance the efficiency of nursing outcomes (Coiera, 2013). To achieve this, the health care organizations must educate the workforce on how to effectively use the dynamic contemporary technology to minimize the arising issues. Effective integration of the social media in organizations has the potential to enhance the overall performance. This can be achieved when various entities with similar objectives are drawn together, increasing the intellectual resources and hence the performance.

According to the journal the nursing community can use the social media for education and research purposes as well as communications. However, the utilization of these platforms must be guided by the confidentiality as well as other concerned professional responsibilities. Major risks involved in the use of social media platforms include permanence of information, the scope of distribution, reputation damage, pseudonyms a well as the misapprehension of the extent of privacy control (Coiera, 2013). To mitigate these risks, it is important to reevaluate the risks involved and observe the nursing professional standards in the distribution of information.

Evidently, social media presents an opportunity to increase the efficiency of community based awareness. The ability to communicate in real time and almost instantaneous has the potential to enhance the efficiency of community-based intervention programs in the provision of the health care. For instance, posting information concerning a disease outbreak in a certain region through the social media platforms is likely to sensitize the public on how to take effective precautionary measures to curb the prevalence of a certain disease. Similar strategies can be used to address some of the primary concerns facing the health care system by creating awareness and educating the public on the best health practices. Ideally, there are numerous advantages associated with the use of social media. Understanding the importance of these tools is paramount in establishing the efficiency in the health care set up. Some of the advantages include fast dissemination of health care information, cost effective, collaboration in the health care system and so forth.

Evidently, social media platform allows users to share information on real-time basis. In other words, all users gain access to information updates almost as soon as the status is changed. This outlines a credible opportunity for healthcare agencies to manage, share information and gather credible evidence of the community health. For instance, news regarding an outbreak of some diseases spreads like wildfire across the world. Classic examples are communicable diseases, whose news broke the internet through the social media (Coiera, 2013). Using these platforms, the health care agencies are able to share details of signs and symptoms of these diseases, making it easier for the public seek medical health in case they are affected. These efforts have played a crucial role in curbing the spread of contagious diseases, saving the international community of epidemics that could have otherwise consumed lots of lives.

Briefly, social media tools are vital in sharing health care information. People willing to understand certain diseases often visit blogs, among other platforms where information is provided. Moreover, it is not mandatory for the client to seek sensitive information from the healthcare system (Coiera, 2013). Instead, learning the clinical manifestation, preventive and management measures of certain diseases enables the community to seek quality and precise health care services. Thus, the healthcare disparities are reduced and at the same time increasing the overall quality health of individuals.

Social media is the best thing that happened to the communication industry after the inception of internet in the digital age. Most social media accounts require no or little cost to register, manage and operate an account. For example, all that a person needs when setting a Facebook account is a simple data plan and personal information. On the contrary, the cost of print media is relatively high because of printing and distribution of the hard copies to the communities. However, the only cost incurred in social media platform is that of writing the content and uploading it. Nurses can effectively use social media platforms to maximize the efficiency of already depleted resources. This is particularly vital as it beats the odds of distance along with those of disseminating information. As previously mentioned, social media platforms are quick and also cheap in advancing healthcare objectives. When used effectively, these platforms play a central role in preventing, promotional campaigns and diagnosing the overall health of the community. Through online surveys, data gathered can also be utilized in the formulation of healthcare policies as well as to improve the overall system.

More often than not, social media has provided a common ground between consumers and companies. Through reviews criticism and comments, companies using customer-oriented approach tend to use the gathered information to advance and improve their products. Similarly, such trait can be harnessed by healthcare organizations with the intention of obtaining such goals. Indeed, nursing practice advocates for patient oriented-services. Therefore, using social media platforms to level the ground is vital increasing the confidence of the patients to share sensitive information through anonymous accounts. It can also provide an excellent opportunity to debunk common health myths and misconceptions.

Credibility of the Source: The journal contains credible information mainly because of the credibility of the author. Towards the end of the journal, the author has been listed as the guarantor of the journal, after obtaining the support of the NH&MRC Center for Research and Excellence in E-Health. The author has also declared the conflict of interest, further attesting to the credibility of the journal. Additionally, Enrico is the director at the Center for Health Informatics Australian Institute of Health Innovations in the University of New South Wales located in Sydney, Australia. The article was accepted and published in the year 2013. This information indicates that the information present in the journal is directly concerned with the modern society and that the content is reliable, and hence suitable for academic purposes. Thus, the paper is used to analyze the sociological approach employed by the author to present the main arguments and the conclusions of the article.

Sociological Theoretical Approach

Evidently, Enrico uses a structural functionalism theoretical approach in analyzing major methods along with the advantages associated with the incorporation of social networks, social media to deal with social diseases in the society. The structural functionalism sociological theory propose that the society is a multifaceted unit that works together to enhance unanimity and steadiness (Segal, 2010). The theory explores the society as a macro-level orientation, which concentrates on the social configurations that molds the community. Structural functionalism views the society as an organism, which requires different components to function effectively.

The absence of one organ affects the entire systems and hence the importance of looking after all the components of the body, and in this case, the society. This notion focuses on the social structures and functions to demonstrate how the society functions. Particularly, some of the major components included in the functionalism approach are customs, traditions, norms, as well as the institutions. These features are compared with the body, in which they must function appropriately for the society to survive, evolve and overcome major challenges. In other words all the components are equally important and they have the magnitude to affect a given community in equal approaches.

Apparently, Enrico has used the structural functionalism approach to present the critically analyze the importance of social networks and the social media in the modern society. According to the author, the social networking platforms present the ideal channel to facilitate interactions with the intentions of enhancing the health care sector (Coiera, 2013). In particular, the author states that these platforms are fundamental in strengthening the stability of the community, with a particular focus on the health care. Specifically, the journal presents the primary ways in which the social media networks can be modified to suit the needs of the society and the nature of the primary interventions.

Consequently, these techniques are the individuals, groups, network inductions and network alternations. The individuals are presented as the opinion leaders in the society, who can influence other people to achieve the desired outcomes. The group element is examined as a feature that is mainly responsible for influencing the social norms of tin a given society. Network inductions and alterations illustrate the channels, in which the information is passed from one person to another. Clearly, Enrico identifies components that reflect the basic foundations of the structural functionalism. As previously stated, the society requires specific components so as to function appropriately. On the other hand, Enrico presents similar components but in a complex manner in attempts to highlight the importance of the social media platforms to enhance the stability of the health care system. Thus, the author makes use of the functionalism sociological theory to demonstrate the importance of the social media platforms in the health care sector (Coiera, 2013). The author proceeds to give some of the prospectus advantages of making use of the social media components to enhance the stability, functionalism and promote the well-ness of the society.

Apparently, Enrico uses the structural functionalism theory to describe the analysis of the theoretical findings of the research. The data is presented in a manner that resembles the basic components of the society. According to the data analyzed, the author uses this approach to illustrate the communication as one of the major instrument of enhancing the strength of the community health. The use of strategic social structures to influence the customs and behaviors of other people in the target society also reflects the structural functionalism. For instance, the definition of the theory suggests that social structures are used to shape and influence the entire society (Coiera, 2013). Correspondingly, each organ has the potential to affect the behavior of an organism. Thus, the author suggests that the utilization of the opinion leaders or the leadership structure enhances the access of remote locations as well as addressing the health care disparities. The leadership institutions are also important in fostering the commitment of the society, where effective programs have the capacity to influence and manipulate the health practices of the society to reduce the prevalence of the preventable diseases.

The choice of the structural functionalism presents the best scenario to evaluate how community health is promoted through the use of locally available resources, reducing the cost and the resources directed towards the creation of awareness. During the pre-globalization era, especially in Africa, information was passed through the word of mouth. The pre-globalization period also forced the communities to rely on one another for survival (Coiera, 2013). Even though this has since changed, the author uses this approach to apply the importance of making the information readily available to the public. In other words, the article uses this approach to support the presumptions that the functionalism factors are vital in the modern society and hence appropriate to incorporate in the health care sector to support, enhance and improve the health care system. Most importantly, the author has outlined various components corresponding to the social functional units (Adam, 1946). The components, according to the author, are applicable in the integration of the social media networks and platforms in attempts to enhance the health care systems. Sharing critical information with the public and among the health care organizations promotes unification, stability and the capacity to overcome various diseases, enhancing the chances of survival of the society, which forms the primary principles of the structural functionalism.

In summary, Enrico suggests that the health care system should incorporate the modern technology so as to enhance the services delivery. According to the suggestions, the social media platforms have the capacity to enhance the ways in which the doctors communicate between the patients and among the health care organizations. With a particular focus on the public health promotion and intervention strategies, the author proposes that facilitating the flow of communication within the society is paramount in improving the health care. Enrico uses the structural functionalism to present his findings and complete the literary analysis to support his primary presumptions. The structural functionalism theory likens the society with an organism, in which all parts are equally important. The failure of one organ affects the entire body. Using this analogy, Enrico proposes that social media platforms have become one of the vital components in the modern society, and hence inevitable to incorporate the basic principles to promote the community health. The functionalism approach has been used to illustrate social media platforms as one of the key factors that can be manipulated to influence the customs, norms and the institutions of the society, with the intentions of enhancing the efficiency of the modern health care system.

References

Adam, L. (1946). FUNCTIONALISM AND NEO-FUNCTIONALISM. *Oceania*, *17*(1), 1-25. http://dx.doi.org/10.1002/j.1834-4461.1946.tb00140.x

Coiera, E. (2013). Social networks, social media, and social diseases. *BMJ*, *346*(may22 16), f3007-f3007. http://dx.doi.org/10.1136/bmj.f3007

Segal, R. (2010). Functionalism Since Hempel. *Method & Theory In The Study Of Religion*, *22*(4), 340-353. http://dx.doi.org/10.1163/157006810x531120

YOUR KNOWLEDGE HAS VALUE

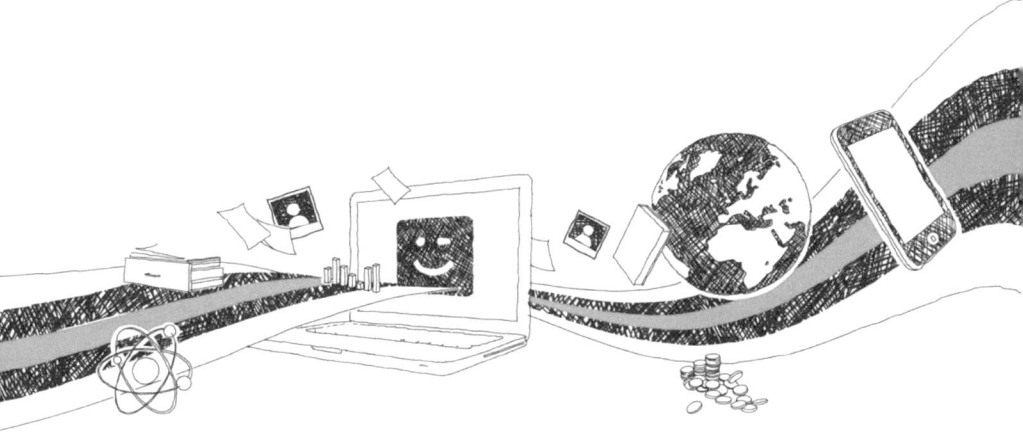

- We will publish your bachelor's and master's thesis, essays and papers

- Your own eBook and book - sold worldwide in all relevant shops

- Earn money with each sale

Upload your text at www.GRIN.com
and publish for free

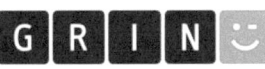